Acting Edition

Ibsen's Ghost

An Irresponsible Biographical Fantasy

by Charles Busch

▏SAMUEL FRENCH▕

FOR PRODUCTION INQUIRIES

UNITED STATES AND CANADA
info@concordtheatricals.com
1-866-979-0447

UNITED KINGDOM AND EUROPE
licensing@concordtheatricals.co.uk
020-7054-7298

Each title is subject to availability from Concord Theatricals Corp., depending upon country of performance. Please be aware that *IBSEN'S GHOST* may not be licensed by Concord Theatricals Corp. in your territory. Professional and amateur producers should contact the nearest Concord Theatricals Corp. office or licensing partner to verify availability.

This work is published by Samuel French, an imprint of Concord Theatricals Corp.

No one shall make any changes in this title(s) for the purpose of production. No part of this book may be reproduced, stored in a retrieval system, scanned, uploaded, or transmitted in any form, by any means, now known or yet to be invented, including mechanical, electronic, digital, photocopying, recording, videotaping, or otherwise, without the prior written permission of the publisher. No one shall share this title(s), or any part of this title(s), through any social media or file hosting websites.

For all inquiries regarding motion picture, television, online/digital and other media rights, please contact Concord Theatricals Corp.

MUSIC AND THIRD-PARTY MATERIALS USE NOTE

Licensees are solely responsible for obtaining formal written permission from copyright owners to use copyrighted music and/or other copyrighted third-party materials (e.g. artworks, logos) in the performance of this play and are strongly cautioned to do so. If no such permission is obtained by the licensee, then the licensee must use only original music and materials that the licensee owns and controls. Licensees are solely responsible and liable for clearances of all third-party copyrighted materials, including without limitation music, and shall indemnify the copyright owners of the play(s) and their licensing agent, Concord Theatricals Corp., against any costs, expenses, losses and liabilities arising from the use of such copyrighted third-party materials by licensees. For music, please contact the appropriate music licensing authority in your territory for the rights to any incidental music.

IMPORTANT BILLING AND CREDIT REQUIREMENTS

If you have obtained performance rights to this title, please refer to your licensing agreement for important billing and credit requirements.

IBSEN'S GHOST was first produced by George Street Playhouse (David Saint, Artistic Director; Edgar Herrera, Managing Director) in New Brunswick, NJ, on January 16, 2024.

IBSEN'S GHOST had its Off Broadway premiere at Primary Stages (Erin Daley, Artistic Director; Shane D. Hudson, Executive Director; Casey Childs, Founder) in association with George Street Playhouse and by special arrangement with Daryl Roth, Ted Snowdon and Jamie deRoy on March 2, 2024.

The cast and creative team for both productions were as follows:

WOLF.. Thomas Gibson

SUZANNAH THORESEN IBSEN ....Charles Busch

GERDA... Jennifer Cody

GEORGE ELSTAD ....Christopher Borg

MAGDALENE KRAGH THORESEN........................ Judy Kaye

HANNA SOLBERG ....Jennifer Van Dyck

THE RAT WIFE.................................Christopher Borg

STANDBY FOR SUZANNAH THORESEN IBSEN ...... Kate Hampton

Director ....Carl Andress
Scenic Design .... Shoko Kambara
Costume Design ....Gregory Gale
Lighting Design .... Ken Billington
Sound Design ....Jill BC Du Boff & Ien DeNio
Hair, Wigs, Makeup Design .... Bobbie Zlotnik
Dialect Coach ....Rebecca Simon
Key Art Photographer...................... Michael Wakefield
Production Stage Manager .... Avery Trunko

CHARACTERS

WOLF
SUZANNAH THORESEN IBSEN
GERDA
GEORGE ELSTAD
MAGDALENE KRAGH THORESEN
HANNA SOLBERG
THE RAT WIFE

SETTING

The sitting room in the home of the Norwegian playwright,
Henrik Ibsen.

TIME

1906.

AUTHOR'S NOTES

My introduction to the plays of Henrik Ibsen came when I was a theater major at Northwestern University in the early 1970s. The versions we read were the late nineteenth-century William Archer translations from the Norwegian. I don't mean to disparage Mr. Archer, who played a major role in bringing Ibsen's oeuvre to English speaking audiences, but his conservative Edwardian sensibility was at odds with the radical nature of Ibsen's work. After reading his translations, I dismissed Ibsen with the cold eye of youth, muttering to myself, "I dunno. I don't get it."

A few years later, at a yard sale in Saugatuck, Michigan, I stumbled across a paperback anthology of Ibsen's plays, translated in the 1960s by the legendary actress/director Eva Le Gallienne. These translations were in a vital, contemporary actor's language. At last, I could appreciate the mystery and insight into humanity I'd been told these works possessed.

For the next forty years, I dreamed of playing the title role of *Hedda Gabler* and Mrs. Alving in *Ghosts*. The odds were slim that I'd ever star in a production of either play. In 2021, Carl Andress, the director of nearly all of my plays for the past twenty-five years, and I were discussing what project we might work on next. He suggested, "What about writing something where you could finally play all of your favorite moments from Ibsen?" I wasn't quite sure how I would go about doing that. It wasn't as simple as putting together a medley of ABBA tunes.

The first thing was immersing myself in Ibsen biographies and commentaries of his works. Not light bedtime reading. However, minor but intriguing figures emerged among the footnotes. There was an illegitimate son from a brief romance with a boarding house servant girl when he was a youth. Ibsen never met this child, but what if decades later, an adult son appeared on the doorstep? I read about a woman named Laura Kieler who had been friends with Ibsen and his wife, Suzannah. Ibsen used the disastrous breakup of Laura Kieler's marriage as the basis of his first international success, *A Doll's House*. What if she returned full of rage over that perceived exploitation? Although Ibsen's wife Suzannah was very much the woman behind the great man, there was little in any of the literature about her emotional life. I learned that after Suzannah's mother died in childbirth, her father, a Deacon of the church, quickly married Magdalene Kragh, the seventeen-year-old nanny to Suzannah's older sisters. Even more interesting is that Magdalene Kragh Thoresen became a successful novelist and playwright. What was the nature of her relationship with her stepdaughter? Was it nurturing or acrimonious? With all of this in mind, I fashioned an original story about Suzannah Ibsen set during the first weeks of her widowhood. I could make her a quintessential Ibsen heroine, haunted by the ghosts of her past and determined to ward off any scandal that might tar Ibsen's legacy. Having played somewhat fast and loose with the historical facts,

I chose to scuttle any scholarly raised eyebrows by giving the play the subtitle, "An Irresponsible Biographical Fantasy."

As I've done for most of my playwriting career, I wrote the role of Suzannah for myself. I've never viewed any of these female characters as "drag" roles. It's always been difficult for me to define exactly what I do. Since childhood, I've been fascinated by the pantheon of stage actresses of the past; Laurette Taylor, Katharine Cornell, Lynn Fontanne, Alla Nazimova, Eleanora Duse, Eva Le Gallienne, and above all, Sarah Bernhardt. When I've created female characters for me to embody onstage, it was not to lampoon or spoof. It was a way of getting closer to these extraordinary women and the theater of their time. I've made my reputation as a comic performer. Therefore, I've laced this play with plenty of opportunities for comedy, verbal and physical, while giving me the chance to play the dramatic moments from Ibsen's plays that have long been my unfulfilled ambition. You might come across some dialogue reminiscent of plays outside the Ibsen canon. Henrik Ibsen has been called "the father of modern drama." I thought it would be fun and theatrically valid to evoke a few of the playwrights he influenced, including August Strindberg, Eugene O'Neill, Arthur Miller, and Tennessee Williams.

Here then, I give you *Ibsen's Ghost; An Irresponsible Biographical Fantasy*. One could say it's the play Ibsen never wrote, his themes and dark Nordic sensibility present, but with the veil of madcap laughter and a most un-Ibsenian happy ending.

ACT I

Scene One

(1906. The sitting room in the home of the Norwegian playwright, Henrik Ibsen. There are no walls to the set, only a free-standing door, a Victorian settee, an end table, an accent chair, a desk and chair, a liquor cabinet and a porcelain stove providing heat. An imposing portrait of a glowering Ibsen is the most striking element. **WOLF**, *a virile, forceful man wearing a sailor's pea coat and cap, enters from inside the house. For all of his seaman's swagger, he also has the sensitivity and virtuosic eloquence of a poet. All his life he has imagined what this room must be like. He picks up a cigarette box on the table and studies it. He hears someone entering from the front door and hides within the recesses of the house.* **SUZANNAH IBSEN** *enters. Dressed in black mourning clothes, she's wearing a short capelet and gloves and carrying a small reticule and a leather folder, which she places on the end table. She enters full of ebulliance, with the slightly mad confidence that the letters contained in the folder will solidify her position as the force behind her husband's*

---

* A license to produce *Ibsen's Ghost* does not include a license to publicly display any third-party or copyrighted images. Licensees must acquire rights for any copyrighted images or create their own.

creative life. **GERDA,** *a pretty housemaid, having heard her mistress arrive, rushes out. She walks with a limp that borders on the outlandish.)*

GERDA. Madame, you left without your hat.

SUZANNAH. I could have sworn I had it on. Silly of me.

GERDA. When you leave the house without your wrap, then we'll have cause for worry.

*(***GERDA** *helps her remove her capelet and takes her gloves.)*

SUZANNAH. Complete and utter forgetfulness might be a blessing. All that matters, Gerda, is today! My dear, you seem flushed.

GERDA. *(Self-consciously.)* I don't know why I should.

SUZANNAH. Didn't Dr. Esbjornsen diagnose that the curvature of your spine might lead to unwanted sensations in the pubis?

GERDA. That humiliating diagnosis is etched in my memory.

SUZANNAH. Was my son here? His presence has on you a *stimulating* effect.

GERDA. I shall not regard Herr Ibsen the younger as anything more than a happily married man.

SUZANNAH. And so he is. And so he is.

GERDA. A gentleman of propriety, same as his father...his beloved father plucked from the living like an unripe lingonberry.

SUZANNAH. Gerda, my husband endured a series of debilitating strokes. His death was not unexpected.

GERDA. Even at the last, Herr Ibsen dominated his surroundings with an intense virility.

SUZANNAH. With his demise, I lost, along with everything else, a conjugal partner of inexhaustible pyrotechnics.

(GERDA uncontrollably gasps with erotic stimulation.)

GERDA. Oh.

SUZANNAH. Gerda. Pubis.

GERDA. Yes, Ma'am.

(Offstage, Ibsen's distinguished publisher, GEORGE ELSTAD, rings the doorbell.)

SUZANNAH. That must be my husband's publisher, George Elstad. You may serve the tea here in the sitting room.

ELSTAD. *(Offstage.)* Good afternoon.

GERDA. Yes, Mum.

(SUZANNAH stares transfixed at the portrait of the late Ibsen. GEORGE ELSTAD, a figure of congenial dignity, enters the room. GERDA curtsies painfully and exits, taking with her Suzannah's capelet, gloves and reticule.)

ELSTAD. A rendering worthy of a giant.

SUZANNAH. One can almost catch him stealing a breath.

ELSTAD. I have just been informed that a memorial portrait has been commissioned to hang in the National Gallery in Christiania and one for the state theater in Copenhagen and an alabaster bust for Stockholm's Valgorande Fruntimmerssällskapet union of scenic artists and carpenters.

SUZANNAH. Is it de rigueur for the bereft widow to be trotted out at each unveiling?

ELSTAD. My dear Suzannah, have I come at an inopportune time? I can return tomorrow.

SUZANNAH. No, I mustn't be alone! Do pardon my morbidity, George. It's thoughtless and self-indulgent.

ELSTAD. As your husband's publisher and you his literary executrix, we will be spending many hours together in this room.

SUZANNAH. For your sake, I wish it wasn't so squalid. Ibsen didn't seem to mind. He blossomed in rooms that wreaked of death and decay.

ELSTAD. The parlor has the effect of seeming off-balance. Is this old building listing slightly to one side?

SUZANNAH. With the walls and its inhabitants turned towards the blinding sun of genius, all is apt to become lopsided. The floorboards, the windowpanes, the servant girl. Long after this edifice is rubble, his glory shall live on.

ELSTAD. We will see him in every future play that lifts the iron lid off polite society.

SUZANNAH. To contribute to that legacy, I have decided to relinquish these letters that have been moldering in a safe deposit box over at the Royal Oslo Bank. I see them as the foundation for a compelling and important book.

> (**SUZANNAH** *enthusiastically hands him the leather folder.*)

ELSTAD. The letters your son recently donated to the Ibsen archive are some of the most eloquent I've read from a father to a son.

SUZANNAH. We're fortunate that Sigurd was diligent in preserving them.

ELSTAD. The letters of Henrik Ibsen are of immense literary importance and I might add, as his publisher, of remunerative value. What have we here?

(He opens the leather folder and lifts out the top letter.)

SUZANNAH. The fifty year correspondence between a husband and wife.

ELSTAD. It's been recognized the role you played in his literary career.

SUZANNAH. His life was my life. My life his life. His victories, my victories. His enemies, my bitter foes. When he found it impossible to write, I gripped the pen in his hand and together we would shepherd his thoughts to that terrifying blank page.

ELSTAD. It's widely known that you were the model for one of his most controversial heroines.

SUZANNAH. I am Nora Helmer. So pleased to meet you. My early frustrations in our marriage, and my cowardice... Did I say cowardice? And my wise decision not to leave him to pursue my own writing, sparked my husband to create a play about a woman who did flee the roost.

ELSTAD. Has there been a playwright with such insight into the mysteries of the feminine brain?

(He scans the top letter.)

In this letter written by you dated November 5, 1877, I see much about a holiday you and your son took in Gossensass, but nothing of Ibsen's play *The Pillars of Society*, which was written during that same period.

(Scanning a second letter.) And here's his reply. Again nothing about the play. Here's another dated, June 1886.

SUZANNAH. A prized jewel of the collection.

ELSTAD. There's quite a bit of agonizing over the purchase of a hot water bottle. And no mention of the difficulties Ibsen found in the premiere production of

Rosmersholm. Tell me, Suzannah, are all the letters in this domestic mode?

SUZANNAH. A rare glimpse into a monumental artist's day to day existence.

ELSTAD. Well, they certainly should be included in the Ibsen archive. To publish, I think not.

SUZANNAH. Not only a wife and muse, I am mother to his only child, Sigurd Ibsen, the current Prime Minister of Norway.

ELSTAD. The harsh reality is that my company is in the business of selling books.

SUZANNAH. How dare you, George Elstad, how dare you slap me across the face with my insignificance! You, a pretentious, ineffectual bourgeois!

ELSTAD. Suzannah!

SUZANNAH. I don't know what came over me. Loyal, steadfast George. It's rather amusing my sudden burst of hysteria. Almost comic. Isn't it?

(The doorbell rings.)

We may continue the debate over the value of these letters when you're in a more objective frame of mind.

(GERDA *enters the sitting room.)*

GERDA. Madame, your stepmother, Mrs. Thoresen.

(Suzannah's formidable stepmother, **MAGDALENE KRAGH THORESEN,** *enters.)*

MAGDALENE. Suzannah, my lamb.

SUZANNAH. Stepmama, always unexpected.

ELSTAD. Magdalene.

MAGDALENE. Dear George.

(They kiss each other twice on each cheek.)

Suzannah, I feel dreadful that I haven't seen you since the funeral. And my blundering rudeness in criticizing your appearance as the coffin was being lowered into the ground. But, Suzannah, my darling, that wrinkled veil with the polka dots.

SUZANNAH. I wasn't wearing a veil.

GERDA. Mrs. Thoresen, will you be having tea?

MAGDALENE. I suppose. I'd ask you to toss in a shot of whiskey, but Ibsen's liquor cabinet is strictly Sven's Waterfront Saloon. No. I'll forgo the tea as well. Thank you.

GERDA. Yes, Ma'am.

> *(**GERDA** curtsies and exits with an outrageous limp, flailing arms and hip twitch.)*

MAGDALENE. *(Sotto voce.)* Oh my, her infirmity has evolved into a vaudeville routine. Is there nothing therepeutic that can be done?

SUZANNAH. The doctors have flung up their hands. I was telling George, it may have to do with the house.

MAGDALENE. This domicile could transform Lillie Langtry into Quasimodo.

ELSTAD. Magdalene, what you are working on these days?

MAGDALENE. The usual. A play, a novel, an opera libretto, a cycle of poems, a ballet scenario and three short stories.

SUZANNAH. Stepmama. You're fiendishly productive in this fifth act of your life.

MAGDALENE. If I am in the last act, I shall take at least ten curtain calls. Rather like when we saw Madame Geneviève Prévost sing Zerlina in *Fra Diavolo* in Stockholm. The curtain calls were longer than the opera.

ELSTAD. *(To* **SUZANNAH.***)* The Prévost Zerlina is the stuff of legend. You must've been quite young.

SUZANNAH. Very young.

MAGDALENE. Suzannah was seven years old. Her sister Elisabeth was nine. I was in my early twenties and hardly more worldly than they. It took some doing to spirit them away for two whole days. Their father was, after all, the Dean of the Holy Cross Church. If their mother had been alive, she never would have permitted such a deplorable excursion.

SUZANNAH. Tell me Stepmama, is there a purpose behind this afternoon's surprise invasion?

MAGDALENE. There is. And it's most fortuitous, George, that you're here. Last night, Mona Lund had a few of us over for dinner. The guest of honor was the extravagantly hailed new novelist, Axel Viggo Rasmussen. Have you read his latest? Such seethingly muscular prose.

SUZANNAH. His book is extraordinary. Every paragraph vibrates with life daring to be lived.

ELSTAD. For my taste, a bit too much masculine posturing and a barbaric lack of punctuation. Zealously guards his privacy. To my knowledge, no one has ever seen Rasmussen. Most likely a crashing bore.

SUZANNAH. If Mona had invited me, I am sure I would have found Herr Rasmussen endlessly fascinating.

MAGDALENE. The guest of honor was characteristically *in absentia.* Mona was livid. Even so, what a hostess she is. The centerpiece of the smorgasbord was an entire vodka-brined smoked salmon. I spent nearly an hour devouring each heavenly morsel.

SUZANNAH. Your favorite pastime. Picking the flesh off bones.

MAGDALENE. But by far the most delectable offering was the gossip served up after dinner about the curious return to Oslo of one Hanna Solberg. Is the name familiar?

SUZANNAH. She was the first of my husband's princesses.

ELSTAD. Ah. The young women he took on as protégées. This involvement with Miss Solberg was before my association with your husband. Did it end badly?

SUZANNAH. I can't remember. While these ladies clung to each word of wisdom Ibsen uttered, they made little impact on our lives. I believe this one was married when she attached herself to my husband. Like the others, she moved on.

MAGDALENE. Well, she's moved back, peddling a diary. A tome rumored to be most indiscreet.

SUZANNAH. What are her claims? Has she invented some obscene nonsense that it was a physically intimate relationship?

MAGDALENE. One would assume so.

SUZANNAH. Well, then she's a liar.

MAGDALENE. Can you be so sure?

SUZANNAH. Ibsen gave unstintingly to these novices his critical judgements, career advice, championing their efforts. The effrontery that this Solberg woman should malign Ibsen and myself! As if I was some weak-willed, acquiescent drudge.

MAGDALENE. George, do you think a reputable publisher will pick it up?

SUZANNAH. His acquaintanceship with these women was purely intellectual.

ELSTAD. The diary will be lucrative to whoever takes it on.

MAGDALENE. What's to be done? Do you make an offer to buy the diary, then bury it?

ELSTAD. I must tell you, she has made an inquiry to our firm.

MAGDALENE. The brazen Jezebel. Ibsen's own publisher?

ELSTAD. We've chosen to have no further contact with the lady.

SUZANNAH. Bring her here.

MAGDALENE. What?

ELSTAD. Suzannah...

SUZANNAH. I insist, I insist, I insist that you bring her round tomorrow. She shall be confronted with her lies.

ELSTAD. We shall see what we can do.

SUZANNAH. Miss Solberg will find in me a most combative opponent.

MAGDALENE. 'Tis best if I'm here when you face the creature.

ELSTAD. That won't be necessary.

MAGDALENE. I'm an old warrior. I know my way round the battlefield.

ELSTAD. If you say so. I must get back to the office. Magdalene, will you be staying?

MAGDALENE. No, I should be returning home as well. I have rewrites due on my new play. Hopefully, this nasty business will reach its swift conclusion. Goodbye, my pet.

(She gives **SUZANNAH** *a kiss on the forehead.)*

And try not to brood. These scoundrels, like mice, emerge out of the woodwork, but a clever trap generally keeps them at bay.

ELSTAD. Magdalene, can I drop you at home?

MAGDALENE. Yes that would be lovely.

> (**MAGDALENE** *and* **ELSTAD** *exit.* **SUZANNAH** *again stares at the portrait of her husband.* **WOLF** *comes out of his hiding place.* **SUZANNAH** *screams at the sight of him.*)

SUZANNAH. Have you come to plunder, or murder, or both?

WOLF. *(With a light Irish cadence.)* Neither, my fine lady. However, the bedroom window shouldn't be left open. Carelessness of that order would never be countenanced aboard ship.

SUZANNAH. You climbed in through a second story window. That displayed ingenuity.

WOLF. I'm puzzled by the décor of these rooms. Ibsen was a man of the theater. *(With a surprising theatrical intensity.)* Where's the drama? The flair? The panache?

SUZANNAH. What exactly are you looking for?

WOLF. I came in search of a memento.

SUZANNAH. Ah, an overly-enthusiastic aficionado of my husband's oeuvre.

WOLF. I am his son.

SUZANNAH. His son? Your mother was Mary Agnes O'Neill.

WOLF. You know of her?

SUZANNAH. My husband and I held nothing from each other. Early in our marriage he confessed that as a friendless boy, taking a room in a boarding house, he engaged in a three-day tryst with an affectionate and jovial Irish servant girl.

WOLF. That would be my old Ma.

SUZANNAH. Those were years of struggle, but Ibsen managed to contribute to your support until you were of age to work.

WOLF. My mother made that clear, and while he lived I kept my distance.

SUZANNAH. And now? Have you written a book disclosing my husband's adolescent indiscretion?

WOLF. Alas, I didn't inherit my father's gift for composition. At fifteen, I shoved off to sea. I've educated myself through Ibsen's work. Within his plays, I've studied architecture, modern sculpture and tenth-century Norwegian history.

SUZANNAH. The glamour of the sea clings to you. Your eyes speak of unsettled waters, saturnine and turbulent. They glisten with the hope of uncharted islands and frenzied ports of call. Or do you merely have an astigmatism?

WOLF. I'm taking all of you in with the utmost clarity.

SUZANNAH. Please, don't tell me what you see.

WOLF. Might you be the lighthouse at the far end of the shore?

SUZANNAH. Ramshackle, with out of date plumbing.

WOLF. *(With a passionate display of verbal virtuosity.)* My salvation is to be onboard ship again, scudding south with the sweaty muscle of the Trade Wind driving her steady onward! The schooner cutting through the fog, her sails taut as the buttocks of a young tart. The surge of the tempest. The foam of the wake. The waves shooting up into the sky with the mighty force of the Sea God Poseidon.

SUZANNAH. *(Breaking away from his erotic magnetism.)* You're here because...? Yes. You sought a memento.

WOLF. With no hope of belonging to my father, I'd like to possess an object that *did* belong to him.

SUZANNAH. An object? Ibsen was not a collector of bibelots.

WOLF. Now I'm feeling foolish.

SUZANNAH. But you should have something. You really must. Ah. Yes. An infant's linen pillow, from the eighteenth century that my husband found in a shop on the Amalfi Coast. The pillow's embroidered with seed pearls in the shapes of stars and half-moons. No, I couldn't possibly give that to you.

WOLF. A personal token would make him seem less like a heroic bronze statue.

SUZANNAH. I never knew my mother. She died giving birth to me.

WOLF. I'm fortunate that I can discover so much about my father through his writing.

SUZANNAH. I wish he could have known you.

WOLF. He would have approved of me?

SUZANNAH. You're very like the men in his plays who have a brutal craving for experience.

WOLF. That hardly sounds like our Prime Minister Sigurd Ibsen.

SUZANNAH. My son is a fine gentleman who serves his post with distinction. Have you been a good son to your mother?

WOLF. I'm away for years at a time. She's content with boxes of candies from exotic locales. I would've been a better son to Ibsen. Often alone on deck, I've imagined sitting across from him in this study and drinking in his theories of life and art. I would have been a devoted son. His favorite.

SUZANNAH. Let me ponder some more on a proper gift. Will tomorrow be too late? What do I call you?

WOLF. What do you call me?

SUZANNAH. What is your name, Sailor?

WOLF. Wolf.

SUZANNAH. Wolf?

WOLF. Wolf. Nothing more. My surname has always been up for question.

SUZANNAH. We have much in common. Am I Suzannah Ibsen or Suzannah Thoresen? Who is Suzannah Ibsen? A lady with a collection of letters covering five decades that today has been appraised as being of little value. Wolf, I shall see you tomorrow.

WOLF. Till then, Lorelei.

SUZANNAH. What name is that?

WOLF. Lorelei, the siren of the sea, whose beauty lures Rhine River boatmen to their blissful destruction.

> *(Before* **SUZANNAH** *can respond, he exits by the parlor door. His sensually-provocative departure forces* **SUZANNAH** *breathlessly to lean against the desk. Pulling herself together,* **SUZANNAH,** *with a new resolve, removes the letters from the box. She begins feeding the letters into the flames of the stove.)*

SUZANNAH. I am burning your letters. I am burning your letters, Suzannah Ibsen. I am burning your past.

Scene Two

*(The following day. **MAGDALENE** and **ELSTAD** are seated with **HANNA SOLBERG**. She is an attractive, composed woman who has dispensed with non-essentials.)*

HANNA. Odd that in all these years of prosperity, they stayed here.

ELSTAD. The house remained uninhabited for nearly two decades when they lived in Germany and Italy.

HANNA. The self-imposed exile. The entire building seems trapped in amber since I last crossed the threshhold thirty years ago.

MAGDALENE. Miss Solberg, I trust that you reside in more luxurious lodgings?

HANNA. My rooms in Copenhagen are far more welcoming.

ELSTAD. I assumed you were financially *vulnerable*.

HANNA. Or why else would I seek to publish a diary of such a scandalous nature?

MAGDALENE. Revenge?

HANNA. Being of service. Bolstering courage and fortitude in others, the young and the degraded. The Mocked. The Wretched. The Aggrieved. The Bamboozled.

ELSTAD. Your strength is impressive.

HANNA. I sense that the two of you may be coming round to my side.

MAGDALENE. Don't be quick to presume.

HANNA. Herr Elstad, you will consider publishing my book?

ELSTAD. Why Stiller and Gustaffson? Surely there are other houses that would offer a sizable advance.

HANNA.   It is of vital importance that my diary be perceived as a link in the chain of Ibsen's canon. You can do that for me.

MAGDALENE.   You place Herr Elstad in a most difficult position.

HANNA.   *(To* **ELSTAD.***)* Your fortunes are tied to the good graces of Madame Ibsen. Do you dare risk alienating her?

ELSTAD.   Miss Solberg, I will say that my mind is open to further discussion. But not here. Not now.

>   *(***GERDA*** enters with a tray of tea sandwiches. Severely limping, she serves* **HANNA.***)*

GERDA.   Your tea, Ma'am.

HANNA.   Here. Let me take that from you.

(She rises and takes the tray from **GERDA.***)*

My dear, were you the victim of an accident?

GERDA.   No, Madame. I have what's called "a degenerative affliction of the spine."

HANNA.   Are you under the care of a doctor? A good doctor?

GERDA.   None of them are any good. Poking about your privates as if you were an open face sandwich.

MAGDALENE.   I shall never regard in quite the same way pickled herring on pumpernickel.

HANNA.   Is the expense part of your trepidation in seeking medical aid? If so, I can recommend an excellent free clinic.

GERDA.   The charity ward?

HANNA.   Not a charity ward. A clinic staffed with compassionate medical personnel. I shall write down the address. It's not far from here.

(She removes from her reticule a pad of paper and pencil and writes down the information.)

ELSTAD. That's most thoughtful of you, Miss Solberg.

MAGDALENE. Munificent.

HANNA. And please give them my name. They know me well from my volunteer work with St. George's Leprosy clinic in Bergen.

> *(**MAGDALENE** rolls her eyes. **HANNA** hands the paper to **GERDA**.)*

GERDA. Thank you. But I don't require the services of a free clinic. My mistress has sent me to her personal physician and forbids me to pay. She's an outstanding human being.

HANNA. Is she?

GERDA. And so is her son the Prime Minister. The Ibsen family think of me as one of their own, and the devil have his way with those that seek to harm them.

> *(**SUZANNAH** enters.)*

ELSTAD. Suzannah.

SUZANNAH. George. Stepmama, Miss Solberg. I see Gerda has served you tea.

GERDA. Madame, will there be anything else?

SUZANNAH. Not at the present.

> *(**GERDA**, with great effort, curtsies and lurches out of the room.)*

You're kind to accept my invitation when you must be terribly busy.

HANNA. Seeing you after so many years, Suzannah, reminds me of the moments of friendship we shared.

SUZANNAH. I understand you're hawking a book with the intent of destroying my husband's name.

MAGDALENE. *(Pointedly offering a tea sandwich.)* Prawns?

HANNA. My diary will shed light on some unwelcomed truths.

SUZANNAH. Henrik Ibsen was flawed.

MAGDALENE. Addicted to praise.

SUZANNAH. Impatient.

MAGDALENE. Dismissive of writers of greater popularity.

HANNA. He left a trail of professional feuds.

SUZANNAH. He gave us an intellectually vigorous theater. An arena of ideas and a social conscience. Nora Helmer in *A Doll's House* has become a rallying symbol of women's emancipation. It is my pride to have inspired this character.

HANNA. *You* inspired?

SUZANNAH. It is widely known that I am the model for Nora.

HANNA. I see you've erased from your mind when I came to you in abject misery after my husband's discovery of my debt.

MAGDALENE. Suzannah, have you no recollection of this?

SUZANNAH. You spoke to me of money you owed?

HANNA. We sat on this very settee.

SUZANNAH. *(Turning to* **ELSTAD.***)* She's asking me to recall a conversation from over twenty-five years ago.

HANNA. I demand that you think back on that day. My tragedy provided your husband with the plot for his first international success.

ELSTAD. If I may interrupt...

SUZANNAH. You are not Nora. It's possible that Ibsen obtained from you some legal minutia, but the core of that play derived from me and my emotional crisis in the early years of our marriage.

ELSTAD. This is getting us nowhere.

MAGDALENE. The subject we should turn to is Miss Solberg's book.

SUZANNAH. Cool heads shall prevail.

HANNA. The title of which is *I, Nora*.

SUZANNAH. That must be changed!!

HANNA. Absolutely not!

SUZANNAH. George, were you aware of this title? You were, weren't you? I suspect you are prepared to publish this abomination.

ELSTAD. I have made no commitment to Miss Solberg.

SUZANNAH. Not a written commitment. Not a final commitment. But you could. You will. You won't. Not if I have to withdraw every one of my husband's plays from Stiller and Gustafsson.

MAGDALENE. Suzannah, George is not the enemy.

HANNA. Herr Elstad, are you accustomed to taking marching orders from the Widow Ibsen?

ELSTAD. Ladies, I am sitting on both sides of the seesaw and it's most disagreeable.

SUZANNAH. Then jump off, George, and return to your office. I am sure you have a surfeit of business to attend to with my husband's many profitable titles in your catalogue.

ELSTAD. If you ladies will excuse me. I shall retrieve my coat and hat and take my leave.

> (**GERDA** *rushes out with his coat and hat. She throws them at him.*)

GERDA. Traitors have no place in Madame's parlor.

ELSTAD. I refuse to defend my loyalties to mistress or menial. Good day.

>*(He exits.* **GERDA** *curtsies in her bizarre manner and exits towards the kitchen.)*

SUZANNAH. Stepmama, we musn't keep you.

MAGDALENE. My day has been cleared of appointments. I am yours.

HANNA. Sitting in this room, I find myself flooded with memories.

SUZANNAH. Distorted and perverted.

HANNA. My husband had taken me to Ibsen's play *Brand.*

SUZANNAH. Your unwitting cuckold.

HANNA. A world of dramatic possibilities was opened to me.

SUZANNAH. Then and there you hatched your plan.

HANNA. I was compelled to meet its creator.

SUZANNAH. You thrust yourself at him. Appealed to his vanity.

MAGDALENE. Suzannah, please.

HANNA. My fatal error was confusing the playwright with his protagonist, the rebel priest Brand. I can set your mind at ease on one point. Your husband and I were not lovers. In a discussion of De Sade's novel *Justine,* he confessed that he suffered from impotence. That does give one pause as to the erotic nature of your marriage.

SUZANNAH. *(Appalled, attempts to break in.)* How dare you imply...

HANNA. Ibsen gave me the confidence to pursue my writing. As a horse doctor with a pregnant mare, he pulled my early stories out of me like a foal drenched in amniotic fluid and blood.

(**SUZANNAH** *and* **MAGDALENE** *are nauseated by the image.)*

Ibsen dubbed me his "little lark," and cheered when my literary efforts were acknowledged. It was the same with all of us. The Princesses. It wasn't sexual activity he sought, but the worship of an adoring intelligent young woman. It approached the vampirish, how he drained us of our youthful contemporary views to fuel each new heralded chapter of his artistic life. I suppose as a girl you were the first to fill this need, until you settled into a dowdy premature middle age. During this time, my husband, Otto, became ill with tuberculosis. The only chance to save him was convalescence in a warm climate. Our savings were inadequate. What was I to do? Otto had an abhorrence of debt. Without his knowledge, I arranged for a loan from a disreputable local character. I convinced my husband that I had earned the money from my writing. Suzannah, you were my sole confidante. I had hoped without asking, you would have offered to relieve me of some of my burden. Stingy of purse and pity, your pale, thin lips remained tightly closed. Otto and I took our sojourn in the south of France. My husband regained his health, but I was unable to meet the payments. The creditors came down upon my husband. When he learned of my deception, instead of gratitude, he erupted in demonic anger.

(**HANNA** *moves threateningly towards* **SUZANNAH**, *and places her hands perilously close to her neck.)*

"You parasite! You carbuncle! You've ruined me! I could twist your neck until your brainless head snaps off!"

(*To* **SUZANNAH**'s *stunned relief,* **HANNA** *removes her hands from her neck and pulls herself together.)*

HANNA. Unlike the heroine of *A Doll's House*, I did not leave, I was thrown out. Stumbling through the icy streets in a state of chaotic despair, my husband found me unconscious in a train terminal and had me committed to an asylum, where I weathered unspeakable degradation. Well, I have survived the madhouse, poverty, my husband Otto, Henrik Ibsen, and you, Suzannah. How wondrous to have found in these past few years a soulmate in a much younger man, a painter of sublime vision, who loves me first as a human being and then as a woman. With his encouragement, I have once more taken up writing, now with a masculine nom de plume, which has unchained me from the condescension all women writers receive. I am savoring a newfound prosperity as Axel Viggo Rasmussen. Yes ladies, I am the man of mystery.

(Both **SUZANNAH** *and* **MAGDALENE**'s *mouths drop open.)*

Last spring, by chance, I stumbled onto the diary I kept during the worst of my tribulations. My lover has persuaded me to reemerge as Hanna Solberg and provide an accurate account of Ibsen's little lark and the amputation of her wings. I shall not be silenced. Before I return to Copenhagen and my young prince-like companion, I shall take advantage of these last few days in Oslo in my bright and tastefully-appointed suite at the Hotel Imperiale. Our visit this afternoon has been most satisfying. Indeed, Madame, I am reborn. Good day.

*(***HANNA*** exits, closing the door like Nora at the end of* A Doll's House. *A dramatic audio effect magnifies the sound in a reverberating echo.)*

MAGDALENE. We handled that with aplomb.

SUZANNAH. We? You were hardly an asset.

MAGDALENE. What else would you have me do?

SUZANNAH. Is that your way on the battlefield? You were as cowardly as George.

MAGDALENE. Should I have tripped her, spit in her face? Pulled out a hank of her hair?

SUZANNAH. You have never supported me in anything. It was foolish to have expected more.

MAGDALENE. If I had made a fuss, you would have accused me of grandstanding. This is your fight. My place was to be quietly at your side.

SUZANNAH. I don't need you by my side. Bitter experience has taught me that you will always disappoint.

MAGDALENE. I shall disappoint you further by refusing to engage in yet another of your attacks on my character.

SUZANNAH. Character? You're devoid of character. You've never been interested in anyone but yourself.

MAGDALENE. Suzannah, I gave up valuable time today when I'm faced with pressing deadlines.

SUZANNAH. You grind out your plays and novels like sausages. Your hackneyed, pandering manuscripts, which expose your limited intellect and grotesque lack of empathy.

(**SUZANNAH** *has gone too far.*)

MAGDALENE. Sausages!!! Now, that does it. Yes, I have committed the sin of being prolific. I write and I rewrite. What do you do?

(**MAGDALENE** *exits by the parlor door.* **GERDA** *enters to clear the tea service.* **SUZANNAH** *stops her.*)

GERDA. Madame Thoresen has left?

SUZANNAH. Gerda...

GERDA. Madame?

SUZANNAH. This house has been cruelly neglected.

GERDA. I've done my best to keep it neat and clean. I am just one person with a crooked patella, a tilted coccyx and a flat foot with a plantar's wart.

SUZANNAH. It's the house itself. The staircase railing is wobbly to the point of perilous hazard. There are loose nails sticking out of the floorboards.

GERDA. One pierced the sole of my orthopedic boot.

SUZANNAH. Well, there you have it. We should each make a comprehensive list of all that warrants repair.

GERDA. An excellent plan. May I return to what I was doing? The day is getting on.

SUZANNAH. It's imperative that our list include the purchase of a proper liquor cabinet. What we have here is not at all conducive for entertaining.

GERDA. Mum, when have you entertained? Certainly not since I've been in your service.

SUZANNAH. Throughout my youth, my stepmother held a literary salon in our home on Friday evenings. May I not do the same? An invitation to my salon would be much sought after. We should inaugurate this resolution with a drink.

GERDA. What's come over you, Missus? Imbibing alcohol?

> (**SUZANNAH** *crosses to the liquor cabinet and pours two glasses from a decanter.*)

SUZANNAH. I'm not opposed to the consumption of spirits. With Herr Ibsen's frequent state of inebriation, one of us had to remain sober.

GERDA. A glass might do me good at that.

> (**SUZANNAH** *hands one of the glasses to* **GERDA**.)

SUZANNAH. This brandy should prove beneficial to the both of us; the rheumatism in my hands and you with...

> (**SUZANNAH** *can't even enumerate* **GERDA***'s various afflictions. A quick toast must suffice.*)

Skol.

GERDA. Skol.

> (*The two* **LADIES** *drink from their glasses.*)

SUZANNAH. Contrary to the myth that my husband was penurious, only the finest brandy would do. I shall be reckless and pour myself a tad more.

> (*She refills her glass but carries the decanter with her.*)

GERDA. Be careful. You'll get tipsy.

SUZANNAH. I haven't eaten much all day.

GERDA. You've barely consumed anything for weeks.

SUZANNAH. My husband's illness seems to have destroyed my appreciation for food. But trimmed down my waist most becomingly. My dresses were getting so tight. I haven't had anything new made in years. (*With startling intensity.*) I was caring for a dying old man. Feeding him a fantasy that he would have in him one more play.

> (*She downs the rest of her drink and again refills their glasses.*)

GERDA. I won't forget you reading aloud to him long into the night.

SUZANNAH. Literature brought Herr Ibsen and I together.

GERDA. And your winsome face.

SUZANNAH. We met at one of my stepmother's soirées. I was nineteen and never felt embraced by her smart set. I remember the sight of him, so vital and robust. The room itself suddenly seemed flimsy and insubstantial.

GERDA. Did Herr Ibsen have that famous grey beard?

SUZANNAH. Not grey. He wasn't even thirty years old. It was inky black and full. A man had arrived. A man. The other guests found the young Henrik Ibsen a boor, pontificating on his dreams of a Norwegian National theater.

  (**SUZANNAH** *places the decanter and glass on the desk.*)

GERDA. I suppose at a party, it might seem out of place.

SUZANNAH. I was mesmerized. One of the guests played a waltz on the violin and we danced. Who would have thought with his stern, unforgiving principles, that he'd be a superb dancer. After we exhausted ourselves with a swirling waltz, a sprightly polka and a savage schottische, he helped himself freely to the smorgasbord. I longed for him to sample everything my body had to offer.

  (*She reclines on the settee in a playfully sensual manner.*)

GERDA. Madame!

SUZANNAH. Ibsen and I were married within a year. He was intrigued and aroused and a bit jealous that, at my tender age, I was a published writer.

GERDA. You were?

SUZANNAH. The year we met I translated the German dramatist Gustav Freytag's play *Graf Waldemar* into Norwegian. (*Crossing to the desk.*) Ibsen was surprisingly bad at languages. We lived in Italy for nearly ten years and he hardly progressed beyond "Cameriere, un'altra bottiglia di vino."

(She refills her glass from the decanter.)

GERDA. Was more of your writing published?

SUZANNAH. No. Mine was a modest talent. Pointless to compete with my stepmother's prodigious output. And Ibsen, his creativity was gargantuan. He would plunge into depths of torment. When he found it impossible to write, I would be forced to…

GERDA. Hold the pen in his hand.

SUZANNAH. Yes, hold the pen in his hand, allowing him to charge headlong into the verdant meadow of his imagination. You see? My words are pedestrian. He would have found a superior metaphor. I threw my energies into his career. I was not above any unscrupulous act to push him forward. There was a theater critic by the name of Wilhelm Brun, who despised all that Ibsen stood for. It was the first night of *The Wild Duck* and we knew that Brun had his dagger ready to rip apart the play. It was crucial that he be kept away from the theater. I had spent days preparing a large cauldron of lutefisk.

GERDA. Ugh. Lutefisk. It makes me ill pickling the dried whitefish in lye.

SUZANNAH. In the spirit of the occasion, I added a few extra ingredients that made it yummy but quite inedible.

GERDA. You didn't!

SUZANNAH. I had the lutefisk delivered to Brun's home passing as a gift from my husband's literary rival, Magnus Nielsen. Picture it, if you will. The butler, Johann, announces that the famous playwright Nielsen has graciously provided Herr Brun, his wife, Berte, and grown daughter, Karoline, with their dinner before they're to leave for the theater. Berte Brun lifts the brass cloche from the dish and exclaims –

*(In telling her story, **SUZANNAH** transforms into all of the characters in her narrative. The characters speak Norwegian. The English translation is not spoken.)*

BERTE. Ah, lutefisk. Hva synes du, Wilhelm?

[Ah lutefisk. Vah-SEE-nesdu, Veel-helm. *(Ah lutefisk. What do you think, Wilhelm?)*]

WILHELM. Så generøst av Magnus Nilsen.

[Sah-shenerust av Magnus Neelsen. *(How very generous of Magnus Nilsen.)*]

(He tastes the lutefisk)

Mmmm. Du må smake litt, Karoline.

[Mmmm. Doomwa smah-uh-leet, Karolina. *(You must try some, Karoline.)*]

KAROLINA. Ellers takk, Pappa. Jeg avskyr lutefisk.

[Ellersh-tahk, Pah Pah. YAH-ee-AHV sheer lutefisk. *(No thank you, Papa. I detest lutefisk.)*]

WILHELM. Du burde bare prøve det.

[Du burduh bar-uh proov-deh. *(You really must try it.)*]

(He starts to vomit.)

BERTE. Wilhelm? Wilhelm?

(She begins to vomit.)

KAROLINA. Mamma, Pappa.

[*(Mother, Father.)*]

WILHELM. Jeg må på toalettet.

[YA-ee maw paw toyletta. *(I must get to the toilet.)*]

SUZANNAH. *The Wild Duck* received enthusiastic notices from all of the critics who were *able* to attend.

> (**SUZANNAH** *and* **GERDA** *burst into unrestrained laughter.* **SUZANNAH**, *drunk from the wine, accidentally slides off the settee and onto the floor, which amuses her even more.)*

GERDA. Madame, I really must go.

SUZANNAH. Stay with me. Please.

GERDA. I must go. I have someone waiting for me.

> (**GERDA** *picks up the tea tray and leaves the room.* **SUZANNAH** *remains sprawled on the floor.)*

SUZANNAH. Is there no one to grasp the pen in my hand? Not a translation, but my own literary voice. Under a male nom de plume. Lars? Nels? Christophe? It's too late for that.

> (**WOLF** *enters once more from inside the house.)*

WOLF. Suzannah.

SUZANNAH. Found your way in through the window?

WOLF. It's the entrance with which I'm most familiar.

SUZANNAH. Angels fly through windows.

WOLF. I'm hardly a celestial being.

> (**WOLF** *lifts her off the floor.)*

SUZANNAH. My husband's brandy has been egregiously ignored. I've more than made up for that oversight.

We've established that you're not an angel. What am I? Not Nora. Nora is Hanna Solberg, also known as Axel Viggo Rasmussen.

WOLF. The novelist?

SUZANNAH. She is that man and that woman and I am...

WOLF. Towering. Magnificent.

SUZANNAH. Rigid. Sexless.

WOLF. Elegantly sensual.

SUZANNAH. Brittle. Severe.

WOLF. Embers waiting to burst into flame.

SUZANNAH. I stopped being an object of desire long ago. After I gave birth to our only child, a visit to my bedroom was as tantalizing to Ibsen as an amateur production of *Peer Gynt*.

(They hear a noise from below.)

WOLF. What was that? Your home is near the seaport. Have you had an issue with rats?

SUZANNAH. A horror I seem to have been spared.

WOLF. I'm told the city's infestation has become intolerable. There's even a woman known as the Rat Wife, who goes door to door luring the rats out of hiding. You do hear the noises beneath us?

SUZANNAH. There's a room below. My husband brought his acolytes to this subterranean chamber for their literary seminars.

WOLF. My father was unfaithful?

SUZANNAH. Rest assured, Ibsen's passions were confined to the creation of a new play.

WOLF. Who would be down there now?

SUZANNAH. My son, the Prime Minister, holds a key to a private entrance.

WOLF. He's there alone?

SUZANNAH. Do you not find it curious the sudden absence of my housemaid, Gerda?

WOLF. Gerda? With her twisted frame?

SUZANNAH. She's a resourceful girl. My son and the maid are rather like the ghosts of Ibsen and his princesses, playing out for eternity the sexual intercourse they never consummated in life. There are other phantoms down there as well. My father and Magdalene. My father and Magdalene. Ghosts. Ghosts.

WOLF. *(Kissing her hands.)* You've sacrificed so much for others.

SUZANNAH. A woman has come forth with a diary that will tar my husband and your father as a plagiarist. My marriage will be laid bare as a sterile sham with me a pathetic ridiculous figure. The diary must be destroyed. The Hotel Imperiale. That's where she's staying. It shouldn't be difficult for a lady of irreproachable respectability to slip in unnoticed.

WOLF. Don't even consider such an action.

SUZANNAH. This very day. This very minute. Gerda! No, she's otherwise engaged. Where's my coat? My hat?

WOLF. Stop it.

SUZANNAH. Let me go.

WOLF. Not while you're in a frenzy.

SUZANNAH. I would make a muddle of it. But you, a stranger. Seemingly without motive.

WOLF. Madame Ibsen, look for another henchman.

SUZANNAH. Prove yourself a loving son. Your half-brother, the Prime Minister, cannot do this. You can. You must! Steal the diary!

WOLF. Not another word.

SUZANNAH. Do this for him! For yourself!

WOLF. No!

SUZANNAH. Steal it!!

WOLF. I can't.

SUZANNAH. You can't. You can't. To perform such an act requires a wild streak. As an artist, Ibsen had it, but you are your mother's child. A servant who accepted all that was thrown at her. I think you should leave now.

WOLF. Don't push me away. The only women I come across are hard-faced doxies who'll grant you a jack-o-lantern grin after you've placed your coins on the dresser and rinsed off your lob in the basin. I'll not go to my grave without performing one glorious task for a great lady.

SUZANNAH. You are a poet's son at that. You'll abscond with the diary? And burn each libelous page to cinders?

WOLF. It will take some planning.

SUZANNAH. Not too much planning. She'll soon be leaving the city.

WOLF. I was schooled by the Swedish Navy to break into far more secure entries than a suite at the Hotel Imperiale. I entered this house through your bedroom window. One might call me a government-trained pirate.

SUZANNAH. My very own buccaneer. *(Whispering.)* I can still hear the ghosts fucking in the lower chamber.

WOLF. I have the means, Suzannah, of drowning out the sound of every one of your phantoms.

(He lifts her up into his arms and carries her off into the bedroom.)

End of Act One

ACT II

Scene One

(The following morning. **GERDA** *is pouring water from a clear bottle into the liquor decanter to protect her mistress. The doorbell rings.* **HANNA** *appears at the parlor door. She's strikingly garbed in men's hunting clothes: trousers, boots, with an archery bow and arrows slung across her chest.)*

HANNA. Good morning, Gerda.

GERDA. Is my mistress expecting you?

HANNA. No. Is she at home?

GERDA. She has yet to leave her bedroom.

HANNA. It's you I hoped to find.

GERDA. Me?

*(**HANNA** enters the room and notices **GERDA**'s fascination with her costume.)*

HANNA. You're spellbound by my bohemian attire. I'm on my way to Frogner Park for an archery lesson.

GERDA. Peculiar seeing a woman in trousers. I wouldn't care for it to be the fashion.

HANNA. In the near future, we'll be seeing women like yourself in houndstooth knickers and brogues. And no more tweezing those pesky hairs above your lip. I look forward to a day when a woman prone to being hirsute has the conviction to grow a kingly set of mutton chop whiskers. Gerda, our last meeting left me perturbed. I do wonder if you're receiving the best and most advanced medical care.

GERDA. It's thoughtful of you to be so concerned. My maladies are a cross I'm resigned to bear.

HANNA. There is a Dr. Leopoldine Graf-Hubermann in Vienna.

GERDA. Vienna?

HANNA. She is an esteemed colleague of Sigmund Freud. And one of the few women practicing in the fields of psychoanalysis and neurosurgery. Dr. Graf-Hubermann has forged a connection between sciatica and habitual masturbation.

GERDA. The very thought! Shame on you.

HANNA. Graf-Hubermann theorizes that onanism stimulates the tissues of the nasal cavity, which can lead to a deprivation of oxygen to the spinal cord. A surgical procedure, known colloquially as a "nose job" might be the answer.

GERDA. I don't mean to sound brusque, but I must ask you to stick *your* nose out of my affairs.

HANNA. Toiling as a domestic in your condition must be grueling.

GERDA. I'll be leaving next week. My mistress has yet to know.

HANNA. Where are you off to?

GERDA. Helsinki. I have a friend who is sponsoring me.

HANNA. A gentleman friend?

GERDA. Why should you ask?

HANNA. Is this gentleman an acquaintance of the Ibsens?

GERDA. My sponsor is my mistress's son, the Prime Minister Sigurd Ibsen himself.

HANNA. Oh, my dear. My dear.

GERDA. It's not what you think.

HANNA. It's precisely what I think. I know the family well.

GERDA. The Prime Minister is setting me up in a lovely flat. And I won't have to work.

HANNA. You'll be walking in my footsteps in the snow. Being beholden to a man of influence can prove disastrous if not fatal.

GERDA. The arrangement is mutually advantageous. My mistress shall soon be rising.

(**WOLF** *enters from upstairs.*)

HANNA. And who is this?

GERDA. A visiting relation of the cook.

HANNA. A seaman?

WOLF. I am. By your choice of weapon, you might be the lad who delivers the venison.

HANNA. *(Amused.)* I'm Hanna Solberg, an author whose literary barbs I hope hit their targets with far more accuracy.

WOLF. You're Hanna Solberg?

HANNA. You know my name?

WOLF. Oh, yes.

HANNA. You've read my work?

WOLF. I have. Anything new for your readership?

HANNA. An offering from long ago, chock full of surprises. Well, Frogner Park is calling me.

WOLF. There's hunting at Frogner?

HANNA. No. My archery instructor has a range on the far north edge.

WOLF. That's a distance on foot.

HANNA. It will be a hike, but I'm a proponent of violent exercise.

WOLF. An all day activity?

HANNA. Should take me until dusk. When do you begin your next voyage?

WOLF. This will be my last day in Oslo.

HANNA. Was it all you expected?

WOLF. More. Good luck with your archery.

HANNA. I wish you smooth sailing. Gerda, if you have a need to talk, you can reach me at the Hotel Imperiale through the end of the week.

(**HANNA** *exits.*)

GERDA. Good riddance to that one. We should only hope that the worst of the archery students aims his arrow right between her eyes.

WOLF. We'll say nothing of Miss Solberg's visit. It will cause Madame Ibsen needless distress.

GERDA. Miss Solberg was never here.

(**SUZANNAH** *enters from the bedroom in a trailing peignoir, her long hair flowing.*)

I'm glad to see you finally had a full night's sleep, Madame.

SUZANNAH. I did, Gerda. I did.

(**GERDA,** *stealthily removing the decanter of water, exits towards the kitchen.*)

Must it really be morning?

WOLF. It's time I leave for the Hotel Imperiale.

SUZANNAH. How do you intend to slip past the concierge?

WOLF. You don't need to know.

SUZANNAH. I must know.

WOLF. The diary will be destroyed. That is a promise.

SUZANNAH. Then away with you. And do it beautifully. Upon your return, I shall wreathe your head in vine leaves.

(She hold his face between her hands.)

Will I see you for dinner?

WOLF. That won't be possible.

SUZANNAH. In the late evening then?

WOLF. Suzannah, the theft of the diary mustn't be linked to you. By late afternoon, I'll be back on ship.

SUZANNAH. Will you be at sea for long?

WOLF. It's a two-year voyage.

SUZANNAH. We can't be separated for two years.

WOLF. Suzannah, we have no future.

SUZANNAH. I won't be like your mother, content with a box of caramels from Liverpool. Wolf, I'm running away with you.

WOLF. Suzannah, the sea is a resentful harlot and won't take kindly to a rival.

SUZANNAH. We'll invent some reason for me to be brought on as a guest of the Captain. Or I might pass myself off as a sailor.

WOLF. *(With impassioned eloquence.)* The sea will rebel and rise up in her whorish fury. She'll open her legs wide and the devil take the schooner that dares thrust in and out of her salty void without arousing the sea slut's wrath.

SUZANNAH. I think we've had enough of the whore analogy, darling. I need only be onboard until the first port of call. We'll disembark there.

WOLF. On what would we subsist? My mariner's wages?

SUZANNAH. Ibsen's plays will support our adventure. Let the ghosts work for me.

WOLF. You're mad.

SUZANNAH. Then I am a deliriously happy madwoman.

WOLF. *(Mulling it over.)* You onboard ship? Hidden in a cabin waiting for me. The two of us making love on the warm sands of Moorea. Your madness is contagious.

SUZANNAH. Hope so.

WOLF. It's lunacy.

SUZANNAH. Could be.

WOLF. Dammit, I'll get you on that boat.

SUZANNAH. Do you really want me with you?

WOLF. I do, my pirate queen! I do! *(Whirling her around.)* The crew is not a refined lot. They can be menacing in their rowdy conduct.

SUZANNAH. I would expect nothing less. Naturally, a pirate queen must come fully armed.

> *(She crosses to the desk, opens a drawer and removes a gun.)*

My husband kept this pistol at the ready and I am told loaded with two bullets.

WOLF. A gun suits you.

SUZANNAH. I prefer it to a feathered fan. (*She places the gun back in the desk drawer.*) I shall carry it on my person as insurance. Now, get thee to the Hotel Imperiale, my love, while I pack a small trunk.

(*The doorbell rings.*)

That must be George Elstad. I won't say a word about our plans. How shocked they all will be when I suddenly vanish.

(*The* **RAT WIFE** *appears in the doorway of the room. A macabre figure, she wears a raggedy coat and bonnet and carries a large bag. She speaks in a disconcertingly mellifluous and soothing manner.*)

RAT WIFE. Have you good people any troublesome thing that gnaws here?

SUZANNAH. In this home?

WOLF. You're the Rat Wife, aren't you?

RAT WIFE. So I've been called. As well as the Rat Woman, Mother Rat, Madame La Rat and in some quarters "Lady Rat-Face."

SUZANNAH. Whoever you may be, there are no vermin here.

RAT WIFE. Are you quite sure?

SUZANNAH. There is nothing of that revolting nature in this clean house.

RAT WIFE. But is it clean? My nose traces a rancid odor. Pungent and foul.

(*The* **RAT WIFE** *steps past them into the room.*)

SUZANNAH. I am asking you to leave.

RAT WIFE. A putrid perfume clings to you.

SUZANNAH. Get out of here, Rat-Face. Get out of here!

WOLF. Suzannah!

RAT WIFE. There is something sad and grey lurking within the walls.

WOLF. One lone woman can go about ridding a city of pestilence?

SUZANNAH. She's evil. *(Crossing herself.)* Spar uss fra det onde.

> [Spah-russ fra dett oona. *(Spare us from evil.)*]

WOLF. She's a harmless old Mother Hubbard.

SUZANNAH. And filthy. The hem of her skirt is stiff with mouse droppings.

WOLF. By what method do you exterminate the rats?

RAT WIFE. I have the knack of seeping into their little minds. Filling them with false visions of nourishment. You see, in this bag is my tin flute. When the petite darlings hear my tune, they emerge from their cramped corners, and scurry after me through the winding streets down to the harbor. I have a little skiff waiting for me by the dock.

WOLF. You man the boat yourself?

SUZANNAH. Why should you care?

RAT WIFE. I have a companion who rows the boat, a disgraced Hungarian circus clown named Gyuczi. As we paddle out, I continue playing my tune and the rats trail after our skiff into the murky waters. Some have held on for years, faded and sickly yet voraciously feeding off the strong. There are words to my melody. Would you care to listen?

SUZANNAH. We wouldn't.

RAT WIFE. *(She sings her eerie tuneless song.)*
WHERE I LEAD THE TIDES FLOW.
A PLACE OF REST FAR BELOW.

SUZANNAH. I told you I didn't want to hear it!

RAT WIFE. Kind sir, I see you're also planning a voyage to the deep. You leave tonight.

WOLF. I'll be damned. What gives you that knowledge?

RAT WIFE. Her chalky wizened face.

SUZANNAH. You dare taunt me in my own home.

RAT WIFE. We all have our roles to play and yours, my dear, is not that of a sailor's bawd.

WOLF. We've endured your mischief long enough. Be gone with you, Veda Vermin.

RAT WIFE. Both with a pipe dream. Sailor, you believe that intimacy with this gentlewoman will bathe you in refinement. And you, Madame, wish to be young, when you're old enough to be my mother.

SUZANNAH. You lie. How old are you, Rat Face?

RAT WIFE. Forty-two.

SUZANNAH. It's not true!

(Silently, she counts forty-two plus twenty and her face registers in horror that the **RAT WIFE** *is accurate!)*

RAT WIFE. Bless you for your cordiality, but I must take my leave. Again, if you should happen to see anything that nibbles and gnaws, and creeps and crawls, send for the Rat Wife and my tin flute will be at your service.

(Singing her song again.)
WHERE I LEAD, THE TIDES FLOW.
A PLACE OF REST FAR BELOW.

*(The **RAT WIFE** exits.)*

WOLF. Don't let the old twat give you the shivers.

SUZANNAH. She's not that old.

WOLF. We mustn't allow her ravings to distract us.

SUZANNAH. The Rat Wife lures the innocent to their watery graves. You are of the sea.

WOLF. Pay her no mind. Forget she came through the door.

SUZANNAH. She spoke of things that gnaw and feed off the living. Memories do that. They breed and devour. She knows of my stepmother, doesn't she?

WOLF. She made no mention of her. But why shouldn't she? Your stepmother is a celebrated woman.

SUZANNAH. She was our governess. The Rat Wife knows of Magdalene and my father. What they did in the room downstairs the night I was born. As my mother writhed in agony, my sister Elisabeth found them... saw them. She was four years old but she remembers. Afterwards, the scandal. The whispers. They follow me.

WOLF. I have no interest in ugly rumors. If I'm to break into Solberg's rooms, I must be on my way. When my mission is complete, I'll return for you. Be ready, my love.

SUZANNAH. *(With a tragic finality.)* Goodbye.

> (**WOLF** *kisses her hands and heads for the door. Just as he's exiting,* **MAGDALENE** *enters. She watches him leave.*)

Why are you here?

MAGDALENE. I was not pleased with the way it ended with us yesterday. We mustn't stoop to such silliness at this time of our lives. Who was that sailor?

SUZANNAH. Didn't you see the Rat Wife? She came to inspect for vermin. The sailor was her comrade-in-arms.

MAGDALENE. When did you begin receiving in your dressing gown?

SUZANNAH. I haven't been well.

MAGDALENE. You're more than well. And that sailor wasn't part of a rodent extermination.

SUZANNAH. The sailor is Ibsen's lost son.

MAGDALENE. From the servant girl when Ibsen was a youth?

SUZANNAH. He came here for a memento to take with him to sea.

MAGDALENE. And you gave him something to remember. A night in the widow's bed. I smell his sex on you.

SUZANNAH. What of it?

MAGDALENE. You fornicated with your husband's son. It's...it's incest.

SUZANNAH. It's far from incest.

MAGDALENE. You've been placed on a pedestal. What will people say?

SUZANNAH. I couldn't care less.

MAGDALENE. Is it your aim to be the object of gross speculation? Is that what you want?

SUZANNAH. What a splendid hypocrite you are. You, whose name is synonymous with scandal.

MAGDALENE. What's come over you? It's as if you've been bewitched.

SUZANNAH. Quite the opposite. The spell that you cast on me as an infant has at last been lifted.

MAGDALENE. Again and again, your wicked stepmother is to blame for all your misfortunes.

SUZANNAH. My father was a guileless stooge to have fallen for the machinations of a conniving young nanny. You should have been discharged without a reference or severance pay.

MAGDALENE. I would've been spared the slander of malicious children.

SUZANNAH. You were seen by Elisabeth. The midwife wouldn't let her into my mother's bedroom. So she climbed down the stairs in search of comfort. And she found you and Father, naked and glistening, in the basement room. Vile. Despicable. Disgusting.

MAGDALENE. There was no basement room. The house was built too close to the sea. You're conflating the memory of that house with this house.

SUZANNAH. My mother died with only a hired midwife present. Where was my father?

MAGDALENE. He was with me but not in the manner you've invented. Let me tell you about your mother.

SUZANNAH. I will hear nothing more.

MAGDALENE. Her death in childbirth was the best thing to have happened to him. And you.

SUZANNAH. She was kind and gentle. Adored by all.

MAGDALENE. She was my employer. I knew her better than her friends and family.

SUZANNAH. Is that so?

MAGDALENE. She was a narrow-minded bovine creature and intolerant of anyone who didn't share her religious mania.

SUZANNAH. She wasn't a sophisticate. Of course, you disparage her.

MAGDALENE. A sensitive child was beyond her realm of understanding.

SUZANNAH. She might have loved me.

MAGDALENE. I might have loved you, given half a chance.

SUZANNAH. You counted on me dying with my mother. And when I lived, you were forced to contrive another solution to be rid of me. I must have been six years old when you engaged that sinister cook, Helga.

MAGDALENE. There was nothing sinister about Helga. She came highly recommended.

SUZANNAH. Why was I given specially prepared meals apart from the rest of the family?

MAGDALENE. You were impossible to please.

SUZANNAH. I can see you in the kitchen instructing Helga to chew my food before it was served, so that it would be drained of its nutrients. She grew more rotund as I withered into anemia. You hoped I would succumb from rickets or beriberi.

MAGDALENE. Ibsen's death has affected your sanity. I truly am concerned.

SUZANNAH. With the strategy of a field marshall you took over the dead woman's life.

MAGDALENE. I was a seventeen-year-old girl.

SUZANNAH. You were never seventeen.

MAGDALENE. I couldn't afford to be. I was pressed into service at the age of twelve. Your house was an advancement for me.

SUZANNAH. It most certainly was.

MAGDALENE. I enjoyed your father's attentions and I was shrewd enough to consent to the Dean's proposal of marriage.

SUZANNAH. You were ambitious.

MAGDALENE. My determination to raise myself above my station should have set a fine example to you and your sisters.

SUZANNAH. You? A fine example?

MAGDALENE. I pursued a career as a writer when it was not common for a woman in this country, and I was successful.

SUZANNAH. Oh, it must have galled you when my play was published and lauded. You never counted on competition from within the household.

MAGDALENE. You had an aptitude for translation. And even that, you weren't able to produce more than once.

SUZANNAH. I gave up my writing to assist the most influential playwright since Shakespeare.

MAGDALENE. Next you'll be saying you were the author of his plays.

SUZANNAH. No, but I was the author of his daily correspondence, composing in his handwriting all of his letters to theaters, students, journalists, even to his own son. He would intend to write to Sigurd when he was away at school, but he'd be consumed in his current play.

MAGDALENE. So you would masquerade in ink as a dutiful father doling out paternal counsel?

SUZANNAH. To this day, Sigurd cherishes those letters. When Ibsen was incapacitated with insecurity I held the –

MAGDALENE. Held the pen in his hand. God save us from that tired fable. Ibsen should never have brought you back here. The place is infested with disappointment. It feeds your delusions.

SUZANNAH. The truth is as I see it, as I choose to see it.

MAGDALENE. There is only one truth. He stole that girl's story. She was your friend.

SUZANNAH. His career was advancing. He couldn't afford to be associated with her. I should know. My childhood was stained by your notoriety. Go away, Magdalene Kragh. We have nothing more to say to each other.

MAGDALENE. You wish to be alone with your fantasies?

SUZANNAH. Yes. Alone.

MAGDALENE. To dream of running off with the man from the sea?

SUZANNAH. That dream ended before you arrived. There is no place for me on his voyage.

>*(The pain in* **SUZANNAH***'s voice silences* **MAGDALENE.** *She speaks gently.)*

MAGDALENE. I suppose I am a hypocrite to condemn you for grasping at a moment of rapture. And envious. He was handsome. Beautiful.

>*(***MAGDALENE** *is about to say more, but chooses not to. She exits.* **SUZANNAH** *removes the pistol from the drawer. She raises the pistol to her temple. Something feels wrong with the gun.)*

SUZANNAH. Why must everything I touch become ludicrous? The gun can't fire. It's a theatrical prop. *(She laughs at the irony.)*

Scene Two

(The following day. **GERDA** *enters and opens the parlor door. She's surprised to be face to face with the* **RAT WIFE.***)*

GERDA. *(Shudders.)* Oh my.

RAT WIFE. I was passing by on my rounds, when again my nose detected something moist and contaminated exuding from this house.

GERDA. You're the Rat Wife. You were here yesterday. Weren't you?

RAT WIFE. I had a most pleasant visit with your mistress and her friend, despite the stench. Has the gentleman returned to sea?

GERDA. It's none of our affair.

RAT WIFE. May I come in? I must insist on it. One can't avoid the putrid stench.

(The **RAT WIFE** *moves past* **GERDA** *and into the room.)*

GERDA. If there was a rodent problem, I would be the one to know.

RAT WIFE. Can there be a hidden room downstairs in the basement? Perhaps that could be the source of the stench.

GERDA. Madame, dare I say, the *stench* may be coming from you. There's no downstairs room that I'm aware of.

RAT WIFE. Come, child, you've spent many hours there. I see a well-upholstered sofa. It hasn't been used for clandestine lovemaking until recently. My dear, you've lain nude on that davenport with your legs over your head.

GERDA. *(Intrigued.)* You're gifted with second sight.

RAT WIFE. Soon you'll be going away. You are wise to leave. There is a rotting in the wooden beams, within the very mortar, that is slowly destroying you.

GERDA. It's just bad luck is all.

RAT WIFE. Let Mother Rat hold you.

GERDA. No, please.

RAT WIFE. Come, my child.

> *(Despite being repulsed by the raggedy* **RAT WIFE**, **GERDA** *allows the* **RAT WIFE** *to envelop her in her arms.)*

Mother Rat is here.

> *(Embraced by the* **RAT WIFE**, **GERDA** *begins shifting her crooked spine. We hear the sound of cracking bones and joints as* **GERDA** *gradually straightens up. The* **RAT WIFE** *releases her.)*

GERDA. The pain is gone. The ever-constant pain.

> *(**GERDA** stretches and moves her arms and body in a fluid dance-like motion.)*

RAT WIFE. The ghosts no longer claim you.

GERDA. Their fingers cannot touch me.

> *(**GERDA** begins moving her hips around. There are no more inadvertent vaginal sensations. She discreetly attempts various hip grinding movements to no avail.)*

RAT WIFE. Is something not right?

GERDA. Well...um...when my spine and hips were crooked, I'd get these um queer sensations. But not anymore. Hmmmm.

(*Offstage* **MAGDALENE** *rings the bell.*)

GERDA. Do excuse me, Mother Rat.

(**GERDA** *opens the door and* **MAGDALENE** *enters.*)

MAGDALENE. Gerda, is your mistress at home?

GERDA. She's upstairs lying down.

MAGDALENE. I have news of a disturbing nature that she will want to know.

RAT WIFE. Does it concern a sailor? I see him.

MAGDALENE. You see him?

GERDA. The Rat Wife has visions.

MAGDALENE. You're the bizarre exterminator.

RAT WIFE. I see the sailor at a hotel on the Stortinsgata. He's broken into a room. Why should an upstanding fellow do such a thing? He's been caught on his way out. Many arms restraining him. He has pulled away from them. Running. Running. He's safe. But where?

MAGDALENE. Remarkable.

GERDA. Mrs. Thoresen, would you care for some tea?

MAGDALENE. (*Transfixed at the sight of the* **RAT WIFE**.) I would, thank you.

(**GERDA** *fairly dances towards the kitchen.*)

Gerda!

GERDA. Madame Thoresen?

MAGDALENE. You're moving without effort. What's happened?

RAT WIFE. (*With the tone of a mystic.*) The house has released its hold on her.

MAGDALENE. *(With hushed suspicion.)* Who are you?

RAT WIFE. The Rat Wife.

MAGDALENE. Who are you really? The face of your youth is floating towards me.

RAT WIFE. My rats are calling. I must tend to them.

MAGDALENE. I know that face and that voice. Mitzi! Mitzi Møller. The character actress from the Theatre Comique!

RAT WIFE. Years ago, I went by that name.

MAGDALENE. It was assumed you had died.

GERDA. Mother Rat, you appeared on the stage?

MAGDALENE. She was in my play *The Prodigal Aunt.* You gave a perfectly scrumptious performance as Freya, the burgomeister's daughter's hairdresser's best friend. (*To* **GERDA.**) She sustained a fine career in low farce. Drama, not so much.

RAT WIFE. It's a depraved profession based entirely on the approval of others and grounded in conceit and ruthless hunger.

GERDA. You gave all that up?

RAT WIFE. My undoing was when I appeared in Goldoni's comic masterpiece, *Mirandolina.* The lusty Florentine innkeeper, Mirandolina, was a role I longed to play. There was another actress in the company of true Italian descent, Giulietta Abatelli, who held a deep-rooted obsession with playing Mirandolina. But I conspired against her, slept with the director and his wife and his accountant and the accountant's Uncle Eilert. Actually, I slept with them all at the same time. The clock was ticking. Offers were going out to agents on Monday. Needless to say, I was cast as Mirandolina. Giulietta was crushed and, within a week, joined a convent in Southwest Jutland (*Pronounced Yoot-land*).

During a matinee, in the middle of the second act, overcome by guilt, I tore off my outlandish wig of black ringlets, and fled from the theater. Why, why, why did I think I had it in me to play Mirandolina? I was about as Italian as a Swedish meatball.

MAGDALENE. That was years ago. Mitzilah, you must come back to the stage. We need you.

RAT WIFE. Magdalene, through my wanderings in the desert, I've discovered my visionary gift and sacred powers of healing.

MAGDALENE. That's all well and good. I see now that my destiny is to write an irresistible role for your return to the boards. And most definitely in a comedy. I seem to recall an ill-advised Ophelia. Gerda, I've changed my mind about the tea. Make it kaffe with an egg in it. And sandwiches and little cakes would be nice. My dear, let us sit in the kitchen. It's far more *gemutlich* than this mausoleum.

RAT WIFE. I'm holding firm. A career in the theater may be intoxicating, but rat catching is far more congenial.

> **(MAGDALENE,** *the* **RAT WIFE** *and* **GERDA** *exit towards the kitchen.* **WOLF** *slips into the room and rests in the Queen Anne chair.* **SUZANNAH** *enters and panics at the sight.)*

SUZANNAH. My darling, what are you doing up here? Get back downstairs! Quickly!

WOLF. That dank cell stinks worse than the brig.

SUZANNAH. Nothing but dynamite will get rid of the fungus. Even so, it's not safe for you to be up here.

WOLF. I shouldn't have risked leading the police to your door, but every path to the seaport was cut off. Well, no more hiding. I'm turning myself in.

SUZANNAH. It's all my fault. I forced your hand.

WOLF. I wanted to do this for you.

SUZANNAH. And you succeeded too well. If you hadn't tossed the diary into the fire, we might've given it back and thrown ourselves on that awful woman's mercy. It's only right that I claim responsibility.

WOLF. That's not the answer.

SUZANNAH. It's done. I've sent for Hanna Solberg.

WOLF. What can you expect from her?

SUZANNAH. She's spent countless hours tending to lepers, the incarcerated and the deranged. Perhaps we'll be the beneficiaries of her insufferable compassion.

WOLF. Whatever the outcome, the diary was destroyed and my father's reputation secure.

SUZANNAH. There will be other books, further testimonies, more virulent than Miss Solberg's.

> (**SUZANNAH** *breaks the "fourth wall" and in the style of the playwright Thornton Wilder, speaks directly to the audience.*)

Some novelist or playwright might conjure forth an irresponsible fantasy inventing relationships and conflicts that don't exist. He might remove Hanna from the wings and place her center stage. (*To* **WOLF.**) Imagine, my love, what diabolical tomfoolery could be made of us.

WOLF. It's our duty to protect Henrik Ibsen.

SUZANNAH. Perhaps for those immortal few in the pantheon, it matters little if their failings are vilified, forgiven or forgotten. Our ghost has won. He always has.

WOLF. You say that with an air of defeat.

SUZANNAH. The dead can't be conquered. Their spirits are in the air we breathe.

(Offstage, **HANNA** *rings the doorbell.)*

SUZANNAH. Ah, here she is, the Norse Goddess Frigga. Wolf, go into the kitchen. It's best that I be alone with her.

> (**WOLF** *exits towards the kitchen.* **HANNA** *appears in the doorway.)*

Hanna, do come in.

> (**HANNA** *enters the room.)*

HANNA. I'm making a grave mistake speaking to you. This is a matter for the authorities.

SUZANNAH. Did you tell anyone that you were coming here?

HANNA. No. A decision I shall rue.

SUZANNAH. Please.

> (**HANNA** *sits on the settee.)*

HANNA. I have a history with this piece of furniture. It's been put to use for scenes of literary analysis, dismissal and now what?

SUZANNAH. A scene of reconciliation?

HANNA. You ask too much. I can save you the trouble of explaining the circumstances surrounding the theft of the diary. The sailor who broke into my rooms was a hired associate of yours. Yesterday, I paid a visit out of concern for your maid's welfare. Your sailor was present and we spoke.

SUZANNAH. He didn't tell me.

HANNA. I assume he was here to finalize instructions for the burglary.

SUZANNAH. The sailor is Ibsen's lost son.

HANNA. You can't expect me to believe that.

SUZANNAH. A few days ago, he slipped in through the window. As you have found with your young painter, this man has brought me back to life.

HANNA. I haven't involved my painter in a criminal act. I returned to the hotel earlier than anticipated to find an uproar in the lobby. As is my custom, I've become friends with the women on staff at the Hotel.

SUZANNAH. Most democratic of you.

HANNA. Your sailor was observed exiting my rooms by Dimitra, the Greek chambermaid. She chased him down the stairs, where she was joined by a crew of international ex-patriots. He had to fight off Kazuko, the Japanese manicurist, Marie-Claude, the French stenographer, Liliana, the Castilian hostess of the tearoom and Fatima, the Arabic laundress. Dimitra's screams rang through the lobby.

> (**HANNA** *transforms into each of the ladies as she continues her narrative. The English translation isn't spoken.*)

DIMITRA. Kazuko, bíke sto domátio tis Miss Hanna. Eínai kléftis! Tréxe píso tou!

[KAH-zoo-koh, bee-keh stoh doh-MAH-tee-oh tees Miss Hanna. Ee-nay KLEF-tees! TREHX-eh PEE-soh-too. (*Kazuko, he broke into Miss Hanna's room. He's a thief! Run after him!*)]

KAZUKO. To which Kazuko replied: Watashitachi wa kare o tōzakemasen!

[Wah-TAHS tah-chu-wah KAH-ree-oh-TOH-zah-kay-mah-sen. (*We won't let him get far!*)]

MARIE-CLAUDE. Marie-Claude appeared: Que se passe-t-il? Quelqu'un a-t-il été blessé.

[Keu seu pahs-seu-teel? Kell KA(N) ah-teel eh-tay BLEH-say? *(What is going on? Has someone been hurt?)*]

LILIANA. Liliana answered: Esto nunca sucede en el Hotel Imperiale. Se debe detenido. ¡Fátima! ¡Cierra las puertas!

[Eh-stoh NOONG-kah soo-SEH-day en ell oh-tell im-PEE-ree-AH-lay. Say de-be deh-teh-NEE-do. FAH-tee-mah! Thee-AIR-uh lahs PWARE-tuhs! *(This never happens at the Hotel Imperiale. He must be stopped. Fatima! Lock the doors!)*]

FATIMA. And finally Fatima ejaculated: Lan yahrub min qabdataya. Alansat hanaa hi sadiqi aleaziza.

[LAHN-yuh hah-rub-mun kub-duh-TIE-uh. Ahl-AHN-ee suh Hanna, hee-uh-suhl-DEE-kuh til-ah-ZEE-zuh. *(He won't escape from my clutches. Miss Hanna is my dear friend.)*]

HANNA. Despite their efforts, your sailor managed to escape.

SUZANNAH. The crime was all my doing. I badgered and bullied him till he gave in. Shall I grovel? Beg your forgiveness? I will.

(She sinks to the floor in supplication.)

HANNA. I once came here begging for help. It didn't do me much good. Oh, for God's sake, Suzannah, get up. Where is your sailor? Is he here in the house?

(**SUZANNAH** *rises.* **WOLF** *enters, followed by* **MAGDALENE** *and the* **RAT WIFE**.*)*

WOLF. In the kitchen reveling in splendid company. Wolf, at your pleasure.

HANNA. Ah, the elusive man from the sea. Mrs. Thoresen, we meet again.

MAGDALENE. I should like to introduce you to the actress, Mitzi Møller.

HANNA. Years ago, didn't I see you in a farce by Goldoni?

WOLF. *Mirandolina* at the Theatre Comique! I saw you in that as well!

SUZANNAH. So did I! You were adorable.

RAT WIFE. *(Triggered.)* I never played that role!!

(**GERDA** *floats in with a tray of cookies.*)

GERDA. I thought you might fancy some fresh marzipan pastries. The round ones are almond Kransekage biscuits.

SUZANNAH. *(Thunderstruck at* **GERDA***'s graceful movement.)* Gerda, cross the room again.

(**GERDA** *performs a cartwheel to the astonishment of all.*)

You're moving with the grace of a gazelle.

HANNA. How can this be?

RAT WIFE. She is no longer a captive of the phantoms infesting this house.

WOLF. They fled and drowned.

GERDA. Mother Rat has cured me of my ills.

MAGDALENE. Mitzi Møller; mistress of miracles.

(**SUZANNAH** *examines* **GERDA***'s spine.*)

SUZANNAH. Your spine is straight and the very walls seem healed. The floorboards level. And the fresh scent of Alpine Azalea. Mother Rat, have you banished the ghosts that ate away at us like cannibals, our flesh restored?

RAT WIFE. The ravenous spirits no longer need you for sustenance.

MAGDALENE. Thank Heavens for that.

GERDA. We're free. Free!

SUZANNAH. Free. As if the sun has at last smiled on a distant fjord. I feel its warmth even as I gaze down at the crystalline water from the tallest cliff. Standing alone looking down. Alone. Alone. Hag, what have you done? The phantoms departed but left me manacled in solitary confinement! Or am I merely experiencing the melancholy of liberation? Can loneliness be but the inevitable dark side of freedom?

HANNA. Perhaps. I propose that there never was anything physically wrong with you, Gerda. Dr. Freud recently expounded in his theory of seduction that repressed feelings of guilt, can take on the symptoms of a spinal and gynecological pathology.

MAGDALENE. Spare us the ramblings of that Viennese charlatan.

HANNA. Gerda, you mustn't exert yourself.

RAT WIFE. Come, sit by me.

> (**GERDA** *sits on the settee beside the* **RAT WIFE**. *The moment her ass hits the cushion, she feels a pleasurable sensation and lets out an involuntary squeal.*)

HANNA. Gerda?

GERDA. Nothing.

> (*She suppresses a smile of contentment.*)

MAGDALENE. My friends, we have pressing business aside from Gerda's groin. What's to be done about the diary?

SUZANNAH. The blasted diary!

MAGDALENE. Miss Solberg, shall we have the Wolf arrested and thrown in prison, as well as my stepdaughter? She is, after all, "the brains behind the operation."

HANNA. Are the bandits still in possession of the diary?

WOLF. It's been destroyed.

MAGDALENE. Would it be fair to say that your chief motivation in publishing the diary was identifying yourself as the sole model for Nora in *A Doll's House*?

HANNA. A simplification, but not without merit.

MAGDALENE. Suzannah, will you acknowledge her as the one and only Nora?

SUZANNAH. Yes. Yes. Call her Nora, Hedda, Beowulf. Be done with it!

HANNA. You and your late husband will not be let off so easy. Ibsen exploited my troubles for profit and refused to help me when I was in desperate straits. The idolators of Norway's grandfather should be aware of his unconscionable actions.

MAGDALENE. Suzannah, did Ibsen express any of this in his correspondence?

SUZANNAH. Of course not. Why would he?

MAGDALENE. In a journal.

SUZANNAH. There are no journals. I can account for every word that flowed from his pen.

WOLF. I thought all writers kept journals.

SUZANNAH. Only notebooks with ideas for plays. *(With a burst of inspiration.)* But what if he did?

MAGDALENE. So, there is a journal hidden away?

SUZANNAH. What if quite out of character, he kept a diary revealing this particular relationship. He poured into these pages his abandonment of Hanna. And his unscrupulous use of her experiences.

HANNA. But you say no such diary exists.

SUZANNAH. Hanna, you will write down all you can remember, the date of each encounter that will prove the veracity of your tale, and I, I shall compose it in Ibsen's voice.

WOLF. Forge the document?

HANNA. You tell my story?

SUZANNAH. Yes. Me. The acclaimed translator of Gustav Freytag's *Graf Waldemar*.

MAGDALENE. But, my precious, you haven't written a word in decades.

SUZANNAH. Was I not responsible for all of Ibsen's correspondence? No one has ever challenged their authenticity.

MAGDALENE. And the many letters you wrote from Ibsen to Sigurd.

SUZANNAH. My son has never questioned them.

WOLF. The bastard couldn't write to his own son?

SUZANNAH. He was busy reinventing the Theatre.

MAGDALENE. You would exercise your penchant (*Pronounced in the french "pon-shon."*) for literary ventriloquism to create a fictional journal.

SUZANNAH. Never with a play, but I bloody well could in prose.

MAGDALENE. George will positively levitate having a new title in the catalogue.

HANNA. Once again, my life is stolen from me by the Ibsens. You people are without conscience. It will be a trauma reliving the past, but I shall write it as a memoir. And then, I gladly wash my hands of the lot of you.

MAGDALENE. Face it, my girl, a lost confession from the great man will sell far better than an accuser's shrill diatribe.

HANNA. I beg your pardon.

MAGDALENE. And as recompense, Suzannah, you can hand over to Miss Solberg all the profits.

SUZANNAH. All the profits?

HANNA. This I find interesting.

WOLF. Miss Solberg, you might add to the sales of the book by having Axel Viggo Rasmussen provide a foreword.

HANNA. *(Mulling it over.)* Rasmussen would have much to say in defense of the young lark.

MAGDALENE. Two male impersonators collaborating on one volume. Delicious.

HANNA. No. No. I cannot have my ordeal translated once again through Ibsen's voice. I couldn't live with myself.

SUZANNAH. Hanna, you won't simply be a source of information, but a close collaborator. Allow me to encounter Ibsen as you knew him.

WOLF. It will be a most dangerous and exhilirating literary adventure.

SUZANNAH. Rather like being at sea, eh? Scudding South with the sweaty muscle of the Trade Wind driving us steady forward.

HANNA. You're seducing me intellectually as your husband did.

WOLF. Something doesn't jibe. Suzannah, why would you present to a publisher a recovered journal that divulges your late husband's moral weakness? And one which would portray you as a manipulative two-faced shrike.

MAGDALENE. He does have a point.

SUZANNAH. He does have a point.

RAT WIFE. GUILT! She must expunge herself of GUILT. She can no longer live with the guilt of her inexcusable actions towards Miss Abatelli... I mean, Miss Solberg.

HANNA. Suzannah, I shall join you on your adventure, but I won't be dismissed as an overwrought harpie.

SUZANNAH. Nor will I.

(*The two* **WOMEN** *shake hands.*)

MAGDALENE. I shall place you both on a strict schedule. We're going to want a first draft by the end of summer.

SUZANNAH. End of summer? Stepmama, you are a tyrant.

MAGDALENE. Suzannah, have you paper and a pencil? I'd like to jot down some preliminary deadlines.

(**SUZANNAH** *motions to* **GERDA,** *who retrieves three notebooks and pencils from the desk drawer.*)

HANNA. I have other commitments. Axel Viggo Rasmussen's next novel is due by the end of the year.

SUZANNAH. Do you seek vindication or not? I intend to put in twelve-hour days.

(**GERDA** *hands a notebook and pencil to* **SUZANNAH, MAGDALENE** *and* **HANNA.**)

MAGDALENE. Deluxe leather binding.

SUZANNAH. I purchased them by the dozen when we were living in Italy. (*To* **HANNA**) If this is in the form of a daily journal, we should date the top of each entry. When did you first sink your coarsely manicured talons into my husband?

HANNA. I wrote to Ibsen in June of 1868. But we didn't meet until later in the fall.

MAGDALENE. You'll have to be more specific.

RAT WIFE. October 23rd. The cusp of Libra and Scorpius. Use that.

WOLF. *(Overlapping.)* You're a devotee of astrology?

GERDA. *(Overlapping.)* October 23rd. That's my birthday.

HANNA. *(Overlapping.)* I wouldn't need to use that if my diary hadn't been destroyed.

MAGDALENE. *(Overlapping.)* All the heroines in my novels are born under the sign of Capricorn.

RAT WIFE. *(Overlapping.)* My rats are responsive to the rise and descent of the moon.

SUZANNAH. *(Jotting on her pad of paper.)* The 23rd of October it shall be.

WOLF. We should make a pact that nothing discussed leaves this room.

(**WOLF** *removes a string from his pocket.*)

MAGDALENE. A secret pact. I adore it. Leave it to the sailor.

WOLF. We'll engage in a seaman's mystic knot.

(*He ties a knot in the string.*)

There. Each of you tie an additional knot.

RAT WIFE. I should like to be next.

(**WOLF** *hands it to her and she ties a knot in the string. As* **GERDA, HANNA** *and* **MAGDALENE** *take turns tying a knot in the string,* **SUZANNAH,** *in a fit of inspiration, is composing an opening paragraph.*)

HANNA. The Ancient Babylonians had a similar ritual.

GERDA. Do I get to join?

HANNA. Your silence is as requisite as ours.

> *(When she finished her knot, she hands it to* **GERDA**.*)*

GERDA. Let anyone try to untie this one.

> *(***GERDA** *hands it to* **MAGDALENE**.*)*

MAGDALENE. Does it matter that the knots aren't evenly spaced?

WOLF. What's important is the symbolism that we're bound together in secrecy.

MAGDALENE. Done. *(Offers it to* **SUZANNAH**.*)* Suzannah?

SUZANNAH. One moment.

HANNA. We're not expecting an opening paragraph fit for publication.

MAGDALENE. A professional writer compiles copious notes before committing anything to paper.

SUZANNAH. Here are the opening lines. *(Reading.)* October 23rd, 1868. The morning was unrelentingly joyless and spiritually desolate.

MAGDALENE. Sounds like him.

SUZANNAH. In a state of terror, I stared at the blank parchment. Suzannah, sensuous and feline, entered the room as if by thought transference. Alert to the paralyzing dread in my eyes, my wife gripped the pen in my hand, as the words tumbled forth from my imagination and onto the empty page.

> *(The others are amused by her accurate imitation of Ibsen's prose.* **HANNA** *proceeds to write down dates, as* **MAGDALENE** *plans the writing schedule.* **SUZANNAH** *is lost in creative thought.* **WOLF** *motions to the* **RAT WIFE** *and* **GERDA** *that it's best to leave*

the three women of letters to their craft and guides them out of the room. The writing continues.)

End of Play